MASTERING THE MIND DIET

A COMPREHENSIVE GUIDE TO BRAIN BOOSTING NUTRITION

AHMED .R

Contents

CHAPTER ONE

INTRODUCTION

"Mediterranean-DASH Intervention for Neurodegenerative Delay," or the MIND diet, is a dietary pattern created especially to support brain health and lower the risk of neurodegenerative disorders like Alzheimer's disease and age-related cognitive decline. The MIND diet, created by researchers at Rush University Medical Center in Chicago, incorporates components of the DASH (Dietary Approaches to Stop Hypertension) and Mediterranean diets, both of which have been linked to a number of health advantages.

The MIND diet places a strong emphasis on consuming foods including fruits, vegetables, whole grains, nuts, seeds, legumes, fish, and fowl that are high in nutrients and are thought to boost brain health. Additionally, it suggests reducing consumption of items like red meat, cheese, butter and margarine, pastries, sweets, and fried or fast food that have been connected to cognitive deterioration.

This introduction to the MIND diet will cover its fundamental ideas, the scientific data proving its efficacy, and useful advice on how to include MIND-friendly foods in your diet to promote brain health and general wellbeing.

The MIND diet is a set of eating guidelines created especially to support brain function and lower the risk of cognitive decline and neurodegenerative illnesses like Alzheimer's. It incorporates components of the DASH (Dietary Approaches to Stop Hypertension) diet and the Mediterranean diet, two popular diets. The MIND diet discourages the eating of foods linked to cognitive decline and places an emphasis on nutrients that are thought to improve cognitive performance and overall brain health.

Fundamental Ideas of the MIND Diet:

Plant-Based Foods: Fruits, vegetables, whole grains, nuts, seeds, legumes, and olive oil are all recommended components of the MIND diet. These foods are abundant in nutrients that are good for the health of the brain, such as vitamins, minerals, and antioxidants.

Moderate Protein Consumption: Lean protein sources including fish, poultry, and eggs are included in the MIND diet in moderation. Red meat, which is linked to greater rates of cognitive impairment, is not recommended in favor of these types of protein.

Healthy Fats: An essential aspect of the MIND diet are healthy fats, especially those in nuts, seeds, olive oil, and fatty seafood like salmon.

These lipids maintain the health of the brain and supply vital nutrients.

Reduced Intake of Unhealthy Foods: The MIND diet suggests cutting back on foods like cheese, red meat, butter and margarine, sweets, pastries, and fried or fast food that are linked to cognitive impairment.

Particular Food Suggestions: The MIND diet focuses a lot of attention on certain foods that are thought to be particularly good for brain health. These foods include whole grains, fish, chicken, leafy green vegetables, berries, almonds, olive oil, and wine (in moderation).

Scientific Support:

Following the MIND diet may be linked to a lower risk of cognitive decline and Alzheimer's disease, according to a number of studies. According to research, adopting the MIND diet may enhance overall brain health, lower the risk of Alzheimer's disease, and slow the rate of cognitive decline.

Useful Advice for Adhering to the MIND Diet:

Emphasis on Plant-Based Foods: At each meal, try to have half of your plate full of fruits and vegetables. In order to make sure you're getting a wide range of nutrients, including a selection of colored fruits and veggies.

Include Whole Grains: Opt for whole grains like brown rice, quinoa, oats, and whole wheat pasta and bread. These meals supply nutrients and fiber to help maintain the health of the brain.

Include Healthy Fats: Frequently include foods high in fat, such as avocados, nuts, seeds, olive oil, and fatty seafood like salmon, in your diet.

Eat Less Unhealthy Foods: Cut back on processed foods, refined sugars, and foods high in trans and saturated fats. Reduce your intake of fried meals, cheese, butter and margarine, pastries, and sweets.

Remain Hydrated: As dehydration can impair cognitive performance, stay hydrated throughout the day by drinking lots of water.

Moderate Alcohol Consumption: Use moderation when consuming alcohol if you decide to do so. For ladies, limit consumption to one glass and for males, to two glasses per day.

You may promote brain health and lower your risk of cognitive decline as you age by adhering to the MIND diet's tenets and selecting healthful foods.

Comprehending the Principles of the MIND Diet

The MIND diet is a set of eating guidelines created especially to promote brain health and lower the risk of cognitive decline and neurodegenerative illnesses like Alzheimer's. It combines aspects of the DASH (Dietary Approaches to Stop Hypertension) and Mediterranean diets, emphasizing foods high in nutrients thought to support cognitive function while minimizing those linked to cognitive decline.

Fundamental Ideas of the MIND Diet:

Plant-Based Foods: Eating a range of fruits, vegetables, whole grains, nuts, seeds, and legumes is recommended by the MIND diet. These meals are abundant in antioxidants, vitamins, minerals, and other substances that promote brain function.

Regular Consumption of Leafy Greens: The MIND diet places special emphasis on leafy greens like spinach, kale, and collard greens because of their high antioxidant content and other advantageous substances that may prevent cognitive deterioration.

Berries as a Crucial Element: The MIND diet places a strong emphasis on berries, particularly strawberries and blueberries, due to their strong antioxidant qualities and link to enhanced memory and cognitive performance.

Good Fats: Nuts, seeds, olive oil, and fatty fish like salmon are some of the foods that are high in good fats and are part of the MIND diet. These lipids maintain the health of the brain and supply vital nutrients.

Moderate Animal Protein Consumption: Because red meat and processed meats are linked to cognitive impairment, the MIND diet suggests limiting your intake of lean protein sources like fish and chicken.

Whole Grains: Because of their high fiber content and advantageous effects on brain function, whole grains such as oats, brown rice, quinoa, and whole wheat bread are recommended as part of the MIND diet.

Limitation of Unhealthy Foods: The MIND diet discourages or places restrictions on foods that are linked to cognitive decline, such as cheese, butter and margarine, pastries, sweets, and fried or fast food.

Moderate Alcohol use: The MIND diet permits moderate alcohol use, especially in the case of red wine. However, since excessive alcohol consumption can harm the health of the brain, it should be avoided.

Important Points to Bear in Mind:

Emphasis on Variety: To make sure you're getting all the vital nutrients required for brain health, strive for a varied and balanced diet that includes a wide selection of nutrient-rich foods.

Portion control is important since eating too much can lead to weight gain and raise your risk of developing chronic illnesses. Be mindful of portion sizes and refrain from overindulging.

Keep Hydrated: Staying dehydrated can affect one's general health and cognitive performance. To avoid this, drink lots of water throughout the day.

Combine with Exercise: Getting regular exercise is crucial for maintaining brain health in general. Include exercise in your daily routine to enhance general wellbeing and cognitive performance.

You may promote brain health and lower your risk of cognitive decline as you age by following the guidelines of the MIND diet and choosing healthy foods.

Food Recommendations for the MIND Diet

The MIND diet combines particular dietary recommendations meant to enhance brain function and lower the likelihood of cognitive aging. The MIND diet is similar to the Mediterranean diet and the DASH (Dietary

Approaches to Stop Hypertension) diet, except it emphasizes foods that are thought to protect against neurodegenerative disorders like Alzheimer's and have been linked to cognitive function. The MIND diet's main dietary recommendations are as follows:

1. Stress Plant-Based Diets:

Fruits: Try to eat a diversity of fruits, such as bananas, apples, oranges, and berries, throughout your diet. Because they are rich in antioxidants, berries strawberries and blueberries in particular are extremely good for the health of the brain.

Vegetables: Give non-starchy veggies like carrots, bell peppers, tomatoes, cruciferous vegetables (broccoli, cauliflower), and leafy greens (spinach, kale, collard greens) priority. These veggies are full of antioxidants, vitamins, and minerals that help the brain function.

Whole Grains: Include whole grains in your meals. Some examples of whole grains include barley, brown rice, quinoa, oats, and whole wheat bread and pasta. These meals supply vital nutrients and fiber, which support healthy brain function.

Legumes: Frequently include legumes in your diet, such as beans, lentils, chickpeas, and peas. Legumes are a great source of fiber, plant-based protein, and minerals that are beneficial to general health.

2. Add Good Fats:

Olive Oil: As your main fat source for cooking and salad dressings, use olive oil. Monounsaturated fats and antioxidants found in olive oil have been linked to improved brain health and cognitive performance.

Nuts and Seeds: Eat a range of nuts and seeds, including chia seeds, flaxseeds, pecans, walnuts, and almonds. These foods supply protein, vitamins, and good fats to boost brain health.

Fatty Fish: Often include fatty fish in your diet, such as trout, sardines, salmon, and mackerel. Omega-3 fatty acids, which are abundant in these fish, have been connected to better cognitive performance and a lower risk of cognitive decline.

CHAPTER TWO

3. Modest Consumption of Animal Proteins

Lean poultry sources, such chicken and turkey, should be consumed in moderation.

Eggs: Including eggs in your diet will help you get important nutrients and protein. Eggs are good scrambled, cooked, or stuffed into omelets with lots of veggies.

Limit Red Meat: Cut back on processed meats like bacon, sausage, and deli meats, as well as red meat such as lamb, hog, and cattle. Eat these foods carefully because they have been linked to cognitive deterioration.

4. Cut Down on Junk Foods:

Reduce your consumption of sweets, pastries, candies, cookies, cakes, and other high-sugar foods. For dessert, choose more healthful options like yogurt with berries or fresh fruit.

Margarine and butter: Restrict or stay away from using these ingredients when baking and cooking. Use olive oil or other healthy fats in its place.

Cheese and High-Fat Dairy: Choose reduced-fat cheese, skim milk, and low-fat yogurt as lower-fat substitutes for high-fat cheeses and full-fat dairy products.

5. Drinking plenty of water

Water: Drink a lot of water throughout the day to stay hydrated. Try to drink eight glasses of water or more if you exercise or it's hot outside.

6. Moderate Intake of Alcohol:

Red wine is the best option if you choose to drink alcohol, but only in moderation. Limit consumption to one glass for women and up to two for males each day.

You may promote brain health and lower your chance of experiencing cognitive decline as you age by adhering to the MIND diet's nutritional principles and making wise food choices.

There are many health advantages to the MIND diet, but it is especially beneficial for cognitive performance and brain health. The MIND diet may help lower the risk of neurodegenerative disorders like Alzheimer's disease and delay the rate of age-related cognitive decline by placing an emphasis on nutrient-rich meals and minimizing those linked to cognitive decline. The following are some of the main health advantages of the MIND diet:

1. Encourages Brain Health:

Lower Risk of Cognitive Decline: Research has linked the MIND diet to a lower risk of neurodegenerative illnesses like Alzheimer's disease and cognitive decline. The diet's focus on foods high in antioxidants, such as leafy greens and berries, may help shield brain tissue from oxidative stress and inflammation, improving cognitive function.

Better Memory and Cognitive performance: Eating a diet high in antioxidants, vitamins, and omega-3 fatty acids can help maintain memory and improve cognitive performance as well as brain health in general. Frequent ingestion of leafy greens, nuts, seeds, and fish has been associated with improved cognitive function and a decreased risk of cognitive impairment.

2. Encourages Heart Health

Reduced Risk of Cardiovascular Disease: Studies have demonstrated that both the DASH diet and the Mediterranean diet lower the risk of cardiovascular disease. The MIND diet is similar to these diets. The MIND diet focuses on heart-friendly foods such as whole grains, fruits, vegetables, and healthy fats; this may help lower blood pressure, reduce inflammation, and enhance heart health in general.

Enhances Cholesterol Levels: The MIND diet limits saturated and trans fats found in processed foods and red meat, and promotes the use of foods like nuts, olive oil, fatty fish, and whole grains that support healthy cholesterol levels. This eating plan may help lower the risk of heart disease and enhance lipid profiles.

3. Aids in Weight Management

Encourages Healthy Weight: The MIND diet can help to increase satiety and reduce overeating by encouraging the consumption of nutrient-dense, low-calorie foods including fruits, vegetables, and whole grains. With a concentration on these foods and a reduction in high-calorie, processed foods, the MIND diet may aid in managing weight and preventing obesity, which is linked to a number of chronic conditions.

Lowers Risk of Obesity-Related Conditions: Adhering to the MIND diet and maintaining a healthy weight can lower the risk of obesity-related diseases like metabolic syndrome, type 2 diabetes, and some cancers.

4. General Well-Being:

Offers Vital Nutrients: The MIND diet places a strong emphasis on foods high in vital nutrients, which are critical for general health and wellbeing. These nutrients include vitamins, minerals, antioxidants, and healthy fats.

Encourages Longevity: The MIND diet may help people live longer and have better quality of life as they age by promoting heart health, cognitive health, and weight control.

There are many health advantages to the MIND diet, but it is especially beneficial for cognitive performance and brain health. The MIND diet may help lower the risk of neurodegenerative disorders like Alzheimer's disease, enhance heart health, support weight management, and add to overall well-being and lifespan by placing an emphasis on nutrient-rich foods and minimizing those linked to cognitive decline. Including MIND-friendly foods in your diet will help you stay as healthy as possible and lower your chance of developing age-related chronic illnesses.

Getting the MIND Diet Started

A proactive measure to support brain health and lower the risk of cognitive decline is to begin the Mediterranean-DASH Intervention for Neurodegenerative Delay (MIND) diet. Here's a guide to get you started on the MIND diet:

1. Learn for Yourself:

Learn About the MIND Diet: Become acquainted with the tenets and recommendations of the MIND diet. Recognize the foods that should be limited or avoided, as well as the ones that are encouraged.

Know the Science: Get informed on the scientific studies that back up the MIND diet's claims to improve cognitive function and brain health.

2. Evaluate Your Diet Right Now:

Maintain a Food Journal: Monitor your present eating patterns for several days to pinpoint any areas where adjustments may be necessary. Take note of the items you usually eat and how often you eat them.

Analyze Your Nutrient Intake: Determine how much of the essential nutrients such as fruits, vegetables, whole grains, lean proteins, and healthy fats you consume. Check to see if your intake of these nutrients is in line with recommended guidelines.

3. Establish sensible objectives:

Set Specific Goals: Outline your intentions for using the MIND diet. Whether your goal is to eat better, lower your risk of Alzheimer's disease, or improve cognitive function, having well-defined, attainable goals will help focus your efforts.

Start tiny: Rather than trying to completely revamp your eating habits at once, start with tiny, doable modifications to your diet. MIND-friendly foods should be incorporated gradually into your meals and snacks.

4. Make Emotion-Aware Food Selections:

Emphasis on Plant-Based Foods: Arrange a range of fruits, vegetables, whole grains, legumes, nuts, and seeds on your plate. Try to obtain as many colors as possible in your diet to make sure you're getting a variety of nutrients.

Make Leafy Greens and Berries a Priority: Include berries like blueberries and strawberries, which are especially good for brain health, as well as leafy green vegetables like collard greens, spinach, and kale.

Include Good Fats: Make olive oil your main cooking oil and make sure your diet frequently contains nuts, seeds, avocados, and fatty seafood like salmon, which are good sources of fat.

5. Arrange and Get Ready for Meals:

Meal Planning: Arrange your snacks and meals ahead of time to make sure you always have MIND-friendly options on hand. In order to save time during hectic workdays, think about meal planning and batch cooking.

Stock Your Kitchen: Make sure that everything in your kitchen is MIND-approved, such as an abundance of fruits, veggies, whole grains, lean meats, and healthy fats.

6. Seek Assistance and Responsibility:

Include Others: Tell those who can help and inspire you about your MIND diet objectives, such as friends, family, or coworkers. To make the procedure more fun, think about include children in the preparation and cooking of meals.

Join a Community: Seek out local meetups, social media groups, or online forums centered around healthy eating or the MIND diet. Making connections with people who have similar objectives to yours can inspire and hold you accountable.

7. Track Your Development:

Track Your Food Intake: To ensure that you are following the MIND diet and to follow your development over time, keep a food journal.

Evaluate Your Well-Being: As you follow the MIND diet, be mindful of your physical, mental, and emotional well-being. Keep an eye out for any shifts in your level of energy, mood, mental clarity, and general wellbeing.

8. Remain adaptable and relish the procedure:

Be Adaptable: Keep in mind that the goal of the MIND diet is to make long-lasting, sustainable adjustments to your eating habits rather than perfection. Keep your eyes on your ultimate objectives and give yourself permission to be flexible and occasionally indulge.

Savor the adventure: As you set out on your MIND diet adventure, seize the chance to try out new foods, flavors, and dishes. Emphasize on providing your body and mind with scrumptious, nutrient-dense meals that promote overall health and wellbeing.

You can set yourself up for improved mental and general wellness by following these guidelines and progressively adding MIND-friendly foods to your diet. Keep in mind that developing a healthy eating habit is a journey, and that each step you take to put your health first is a positive one.

MIND Recipes and Dinner Suggestions

Including tasty MIND diet recipes and meal ideas in your everyday routine is a great approach to promote mental health and general wellbeing. Here are some wholesome and delectable recipes to get you started:

For breakfast:

Berry Smoothie with Spinach:

For a nutrient-rich and refreshing breakfast, blend spinach, mixed berries (strawberries, blueberries, and raspberries), Greek yogurt, almond milk, and a tablespoon of crushed flaxseed.

Toast with avocado and whole grain bread:

Add sliced cherry tomatoes, mashed avocado, feta cheese, and a splash of olive oil on the top of whole grain toast. For an extra boost of antioxidants, serve with a side of mixed berries.

Lunch:

Mediterranean Salad with Chickpeas:

In bowl, mix together chickpeas, sliced cucumber, red onion, cherry tomatoes, Kalamata olives, and crumbled feta cheese. For a tasty and filling salad, toss with a dressing of olive oil, lemon juice, garlic, and dried oregano.

Bell peppers stuffed with quinoa:

Prepare the quinoa following the directions on the box, then combine it with chopped cilantro, diced tomatoes, diced bell peppers, diced corn, and a squeeze of lime juice. Bake the filled bell peppers in halves until they are soft.

Dinner is

Salmon baked with dill and lemon:

Season salmon fillets with salt, pepper, lemon juice, and fresh dill before placing them on a baking pan. Bake until well cooked and tender. For a well-balanced dinner, serve with quinoa and steamed broccoli.

Stir-fried vegetables with tofu:

In a wok, stir-fry tofu, broccoli, bell peppers, snap peas, carrots, and mushrooms using a concoction of sesame oil, soy sauce, and ginger. Serve with cauliflower rice or brown rice for a filling, vegetable-rich supper.

Munchies:

Berries and Nuts Combined:

For a filling and healthful snack full of antioxidants and beneficial fats, try a handful of mixed nuts (almonds, walnuts, and cashews) with a portion of fresh berries.

Greek Yogurt Concession:

Greek yogurt layered with granola, sliced bananas, and honey for a tasty, high-protein snack that fulfills sweet tooths and delivers vital nutrients.

Sweets:

Covered in Dark Chocolate Strawberries:

Fresh strawberries should be dipped in molten dark chocolate and cooled on a baking sheet covered with parchment paper until the chocolate solidifies. Savor this guilt-free, antioxidant-rich treat.

Apples Baked with Cinnamon:

After coreing the apples, stuff the interior with a blend of oats, chopped almonds, cinnamon, and maple syrup. For a pleasant and wholesome dessert option, bake the apples until they are soft.

Drink:

Lemon-infused green tea:

Squeeze some fresh lemon juice into your cup of green tea for a revitalizing, antioxidant-rich beverage that promotes mental clarity and general wellbeing.

You may incorporate tasty and nutritious foods into your everyday routine by starting with these MIND diet-friendly dishes and meal ideas. Please use your imagination to modify these recipes to fit your dietary requirements and taste preferences. Always remember to emphasize balance, diversity, and eating wholesome meals that promote the best possible brain function and general wellness.

Advice for Meal Planning and Grocery Shopping

Effective meal planning and grocery shopping can help you stick to the MIND diet and make healthier decisions. The following advice can help you prepare meals more quickly and shop for groceries:

Tips for Grocery Shopping:

Plan Ahead: Make a weekly meal plan before you go grocery shopping. Make a list of the ingredients you'll need for the meals you have planned and take stock of what you already have in your fridge and pantry.

Follow the Perimeter: Fresh vegetables, lean meats, dairy products, and whole grains are typically found around the perimeter of grocery stores. Since these categories typically contain healthier selections, try to stock your shop mostly with items from them.

Select Colorful Produce: To make sure you're getting a wide range of nutrients and antioxidants, try to include a variety of fruits and vegetables in different hues. When possible, choose seasonal, fresh produce.

Examine Labels: Pay close attention to the nutrition information on packaged items. Select goods with low levels of harmful fats, salt, and added sugars. Seek out whole grain options and make sure there are no additives or allergies present.

Stock Up on Staples: Whole grains (brown rice, quinoa, oats), legumes (beans, lentils), nuts, seeds, olive oil, herbs, and spices are examples of staples that are good for the MIND diet. These are the main ingredients in a lot of healthy recipes.

Pick Lean Proteins: Opt for protein sources that are low in fat, such as fish, chicken, tofu, tempeh, beans, and lentils. When purchasing, try to find organic or grass-fed choices. Try to include omega-3 fatty acid-rich fish at least twice a week.

CHAPTER THREE

Reduce Your Consumption of Processed Foods: Because processed and packaged foods frequently include extra sugars, bad fats, and preservatives, reduce the amount of these items you buy. Whenever feasible, choose whole, less processed meals instead.

Tips for Preparing Meals:

Set Aside Time: Make a weekly food prep schedule that includes a particular day or time. This might occur on the weekend or at a time during the week when you're not as busy. Set aside time in your calendar to concentrate on making meals and snacks for the following several days.

Cook in bulk: Make huge quantities of basic items like grains, meats, and veggies so you can utilize them for several meals a week. For quick and simple meal assembly, cook grains like quinoa or brown rice in bulk and keep them in the freezer or refrigerator.

Prepare Produce: To make snacking and meal preparation easier, wash, chop, and portion fruits and vegetables. To ensure they are ready when you need them, keep them in the refrigerator in airtight containers or resealable bags.

Divide and Conquer: Prepare meals and snacks ahead of time by portioning them out using divided containers. This might facilitate grabbing a healthy meal on hectic days and help avoid overindulging.

Try Out Some Make-Ahead Recipes: Look at recipes that can be prepared in advance and frozen for later meals. Soups, stews, casseroles, and salads can be portioned out for easy weekday lunches or dinners and taste even better the next day.

Remain Organized: To expedite the meal preparation process, keep your kitchen stocked with necessary cooking tools, utensils, and storage containers. To prevent confusion, clearly mark containers with the contents and date.

Remain Adaptable: Although meal planning can save time and facilitate healthy eating, it's crucial to remain adaptable and adjust to your preferences and schedule. Try out new recipes and make any necessary adjustments to your meal plan without fear.

You may streamline the MIND diet and increase your chances of sticking to your wellness and health objectives by implementing these grocery shopping and meal preparation strategies into your daily routine. Always make a plan, give nutrient-rich foods top priority, and identify the tactics that best suit your tastes and way of life.

Eating Out and Social Events

While following the MIND diet when dining out or at social events might provide special obstacles, it is feasible to make healthy choices and stick to the plan with a little planning and flexibility. The following advice can help you manage eating out and social gatherings while adhering to the MIND diet:

Eating Outside:

Investigate Restaurants in Advance: Check out the menu online to find MIND diet-friendly options before deciding on a restaurant. These days, a lot of establishments have healthier options or even provide customized diet menus upon request.

Make Sensible Choices: Select meals that are high in whole grains, healthy fats, lean proteins (such grilled chicken or fish), and veggies. Instead of frying or overly sauced food, choose for dishes that are steamed, grilled, baked, or roasted.

Ask for Modifications: Do not hesitate to request changes to accommodate your dietary requirements. For instance, request whole grain options for bread or pasta, ask for dressing on the side, or swap fries for steamed veggies or a side salad.

Control servings: Since restaurant servings are frequently greater than necessary, you might want to order an appetizer instead of your main course or split an entree with a dining partner. As an alternative, order a box to go and divide your meal in half before you begin.

Limit Alcohol Consumption: Beverages with alcohol have a lot of calories and can affect your judgment when it comes to what to eat. If you decide to drink, choose for lighter options like wine or spirits combined with soda water and drink in moderation.

Social Events:

Bring a dish: Offer to bring a food that fits the MIND diet to share if you're going to a potluck or other gathering. This guarantees that you'll always have at least one nutritious option on hand and helps others learn about eating healthfully without compromising taste.

Practice Portion Control: Watch how much food is served during social gatherings if there are buffets or appetizer spreads. Try not to overindulge. Make use of smaller dishes and arrange a variety of nutrient-dense items on them.

Be Aware of Mindless Eating: Recognize your hunger signs and refrain from mindlessly grabbing unhealthy snacks just because they're around. Rather, concentrate on socializing and conversing with people when you're not at the dinner table.

Remain Hydrated: Throughout the celebration, sipping water can help you stay hydrated and possibly avoid overindulging. Drink water in between alcoholic beverages to help you pace yourself and stay under the recommended calorie intake.

Don't Worry About Occasional Indulgences: It's acceptable to indulge in sweets and pastries occasionally during social gatherings. Recall that the MIND diet focuses on overall dietary habits, so as long as you resume healthy eating after a single meal or snack, your progress won't be hampered.

Engage in Mindful Eating:

Slow Down: Give each bite of your food careful attention, savoring its aromas and textures. By eating gradually, you can prevent overeating by allowing your brain to register sensations of fullness.

Pay heed to your body's signals of hunger and fullness by listening to it. Even if there is food left on your plate, you should stop eating when you are satisfied.

Use All of Your Senses: Take note of the flavors, colors, and odors of the food you're consuming.

Using all of your senses when dining can improve the occasion and encourage mindful eating.

You may negotiate eating out and social gatherings while adhering to the MIND diet's tenets by using these tactics and advice. Keep in mind to make thoughtful decisions that promote your health and well-being while keeping an emphasis on moderation, balance, and socializing.

Including Exercise and Physical Activity

Exercising and engaging in regular physical activity are crucial for overall health and well-being, and they support the nutritional guidelines of the MIND diet. The following advice can help you make physical activity a part of your daily routine:

Select Pleasure-Seeking Activities:

Find What You Love: Try out a variety of physical activities to see which ones you enjoy the most. Whether it's swimming, dancing, cycling, walking, or sports, pick pursuits that bring you joy and fulfillment.

Mix It Up: Maintaining motivation and avoiding boredom require variety. To keep things fresh and push your body in novel ways, switch up your exercise routines.

Establish sensible objectives:

Start Gradually: Whether you're new to exercising or are coming back after a break, set small initial goals and build up to a more intense and longer workout over time. According to health guidelines, try to get at least 150 minutes a week of moderate-intensity aerobic activity or 75 minutes of vigorous-intensity activity.

Establish SMART goals: These are objectives that are Time-bound, Relevant, Measurable, Achievable, and Specific. As an illustration, set goals like walking for thirty minutes five days a week or finishing a specific amount of strength training sessions each week.

Develop a Habit of It:

Plan Frequent Workouts: Make time for exercise on your calendar just like you would any other important appointment. Establishing a long-lasting workout habit requires consistency.

Establish a Routine: Work out at the same time every day or week to establish a regular fitness schedule. Maintaining your fitness goals is much easier when you are consistent, since it helps to strengthen the habit.

Keep Moving During the Day:

Including Movement: Seek out chances to include exercise in your everyday schedule. Choose to walk or cycle instead of drive small distances, use the stairs instead of the elevator, and take pauses at work to stand up and stretch.

Break Up Sitting Time: Try to get up and move about a few times during the day if your job requires you to sit a lot. Make a note to take quick pauses from your activities every hour.

Remain Inspired:

Find a Workout Partner: To make exercises more fun and to hold each other accountable, work out with a friend or family member. A exercise partner can offer encouragement, support, and incentive.

Monitor Your Development: Make a note of the length, level of difficulty, and nature of each exercise session as you go. Keeping track of your development helps keep you inspired and allow you to recognize your progress.

Pay Attention to Your Body:

Listen to Your Body: Observe your physical sensations both during and following physical activity. Adjust your exercise regimen or get advice from a medical professional if you feel pain or discomfort.

Rest and Recover: Give your body time to relax and heal in between training sessions. Include rest days in your regimen to avoid overtraining and lower your chance of becoming hurt.

Consult a Professional:

Speak with a Fitness expert: You should think about speaking with a licensed personal trainer or fitness expert if you're not sure where to begin or how to create an exercise routine. They can evaluate your level of fitness, assist you in setting objectives, and design a customized workout regimen.

Think About Exercise Classes or Programs: Signing up for a group fitness class or program can help you stay motivated, structured, and connected to others. Choose a class—dance, yoga, Pilates, HIIT, or whatever—that fits your hobbies and fitness objectives.

You may boost general brain health and cognitive performance as well as the advantages of the MIND diet by including regular exercise and physical activity into your routine. Always remember to pick enjoyable hobbies, make it a habit, set reasonable objectives, keep active all day, maintain motivation, pay attention to your body, and get help from a professional when necessary. You can reap the many advantages of a balanced approach to diet and exercise with perseverance and commitment.

Tracking Development and Making Modifications

Following the MIND diet is just one component of a health and wellness journey; another is keeping track of your progress and making necessary adjustments. The following advice will help you keep a close eye on your development and make the required corrections as you go:

Tracking Development:

Maintain a Food Diary: Record everything you eat, including meals, snacks, serving sizes, and any times you stray from the MIND diet plan.

This can assist you in seeing trends, monitoring your diet compliance, and identifying problem areas.

Monitor Your Symptoms: As you adhere to the MIND diet, take note of your physical, mental, and emotional well-being. Keep track of any changes in your general well-being, energy levels, mood, digestion, or cognitive function.

Track Weight and Body Measurements: If controlling your weight is your aim, weigh yourself frequently and keep an eye on other data like your waist circumference, body fat percentage, and other physical characteristics. Remember that improvement might not always show up on the scale, and give equal weight to successes that don't appear on the scale.

Evaluate Cognitive Function: To track alterations in cognitive function over time, take into account cognitive evaluations or memory tests. These can offer insightful information on how well the MIND diet supports cognitive function and brain health.

Use Technology: To keep an eye on your food intake, physical activity, sleep habits, and other health parameters, use apps, wearable fitness trackers, or internet tools. You may monitor your progress and maintain motivation with the aid of these tools, which can offer insightful statistics.

Making Modifications:

Examine Your Food Record: Continually examine your food record to find any instances in which you might not be adhering to the MIND diet recommendations or overindulging in less nutritious items. Seek out trends and brainstorm ways to get better.

Evaluate Your Objectives: Continually review your wellness and health objectives to make sure they are reasonable, attainable, and in line with your present priorities. As your circumstances, tastes, or health change, make the necessary adjustments to your goals.

Speak with a Healthcare Professional: If you're having difficulties or setbacks, you might want to get advice from a nutritionist, registered dietitian, or other healthcare provider who can give you with individualized advice and assistance. They can assist you in locating possible obstacles, taking care of dietary deficits, and modifying your diet and way of life as needed.

Try Different Modifications: To better fit your unique requirements and tastes, don't be afraid to try different versions of the MIND diet. This can entail modifying meal schedules, portion sizes, food pairings, or adding fresh recipes and ingredients.

Remain Adaptable: It's crucial to remain flexible and adaptable because dietary habits and health objectives can change over time. Accept the process of self-discovery and be open to changing as you get more insight into what suits you.

Celebrate Your Progress: No matter how tiny, acknowledge and honor your accomplishments. Acknowledge your progress and significant turning points along the way, and make use of them as inspiration to keep going on your MIND diet.

You may maximize the benefits of the MIND diet and promote your long-term health and well-being by keeping a close eye on your progress, paying attention to your body's signals, and making any adjustments. Recall that development requires tenacity, patience, and time, so maintain your commitment to your objectives and have faith in the process.

Summary

In conclusion, by emphasizing nutrient-rich meals that are good for the body and the mind, the MIND diet is a viable strategy for promoting brain health and cognitive performance. The MIND diet offers a workable framework for maintaining optimal brain health by placing an emphasis on entire foods such fruits, vegetables, whole grains, lean proteins, and healthy fats while avoiding intake of processed foods, sugary snacks, and unhealthy fats.

We've covered the fundamentals of the MIND diet in this book, including its focus on particular foods and nutrients that are shown to improve cognitive performance and lower the risk of neurodegenerative illnesses like Alzheimer's disease. We've also talked about how to overcome obstacles like eating out and social gatherings, include exercise and physical activity into your daily routine, and maximize the benefits of the MIND diet.

We've also included advice on how to track your progress, make any modifications, and maintain motivation while following the MIND diet. The MIND diet offers a flexible and sustainable approach to healthy eating that can be customized to your unique preferences and lifestyle, whether your goals are to support cognitive health, enhance general well-being, or lower your risk of developing chronic diseases.

Balance and consistency are essential in every eating plan. You may feed your body and brain for maximum health and longevity by adhering to the MIND diet's tenets and gradually, sustainably altering your eating habits. Always emphasize nutrient-dense foods, maintain an active lifestyle, engage in mindfulness exercises, and ask medical professionals or qualified dietitians for assistance when necessary.

By means of perseverance, awareness, and self-nurturing, you can use the potential of the MIND diet to bolster your mental well-being and lead a lively, satisfying existence. Cheers to fueling your body and mind for enduring health and energy.

THE END